MW00889516

Made in the USA
Columbia, SC
21 July 2024

39078710R00057